THE

CHOLESTEROL

REPORT

**Everything You've Been Told
About Cholesterol Is *Wrong!***

By Dr. David Miller

Intended Use Statement

The content of this book is intended for information purposes only. The medical information in this book is intended as general information only and should not be used in any way to diagnose, treat, cure, or prevent any disease. The goal of this book is to present nutritionally significant information and offer suggestions for nutritional support and health maintenance.

It is the sole responsibility of the user of this information to comply with all local and federal laws regarding the use of such information.

Do you really want to know the truth behind the cholesterol misinformation campaign? I will warn you that it may make you extremely upset. Let's look at some of the myths that I will try to dispel:

- ✓ Eating a low cholesterol diet reduces blood cholesterol
- ✓ Eating fat causes high cholesterol
- ✓ High cholesterol causes coronary artery disease

Let me make this crystal clear from the start. Cholesterol is an essential substance - without it you will die! All your cell membranes contain cholesterol for proper permeability and to provide membrane stability. Over 8% of the brain's solid weight is cholesterol. Cholesterol levels that are too low will lead to poor cell membrane integrity which means they will not be able to function properly and lead to disease.

The cholesterol that is tested on a blood test are lipoproteins - a combination of fats and a carrier protein which function like a taxi cab since fats don't dissolve well in blood. These are the so-called low density lipoproteins or LDLs and high density lipoproteins or HDLs. You may have heard that LDLs are considered 'bad' cholesterol and that HDL is considered 'good' cholesterol. The truth is, there is no 'good' and 'bad' cholesterol. LDL particles come in many sizes and large LDL particles are not a problem. Only the small dense LDL particle fragments can potentially be a problem, because they can squeeze through the lining of the arteries and if they oxidize (otherwise known as turning rancid) they can cause damage and inflammation. This is true for ANY fat in the body, which when oxidized can create inflammation from what are called lipid peroxides. There are also different size HDL particles which have different risks associated depending on particle size. LDLs and HDLs just ferry cholesterol in different directions. LDL happens to take cholesterol to the tissues. HDL takes cholesterol from your body's tissues and arteries, and brings it back to your liver to recycle it for other tissues needs.

How did this whole cholesterol and saturated fat theory start? One of the most notable figures in this drama was University of Minnesota researcher Dr. Ancel Keys. In the 1950's his analysis claimed that there was a link between dietary fats and coronary artery disease. What Dr. Keys didn't tell us was that he selectively analyzed information from six countries to 'prove' his connection, rather than using all the data available at the time (which was actually 22 countries). He, in essence, picked the countries that would support his hypothesis. Government agencies picked up on Dr. Keys association of high fat/cholesterol and heart disease theory and began bombarding the public with the advice that has contributed to the diabetes and obesity epidemics we have today: eat a low fat diet!

Another landmark study in this controversy was the famous Framingham Study begun in 1948 and was conducted over a fourteen year period. However, the authors of the study actually stated, "For each 1mg/dl **drop** in cholesterol there was an 11% **increase** in coronary and total mortality". So really what the study said was a drop in cholesterol = increased mortality. That wasn't the take home message that most scientists were telling us. Furthermore:

In the 30 year follow-up of the Framingham population for instance, high cholesterol was not predictive at all after the age of 47, and those whose cholesterol went down had the highest risk of having a heart attack.

Back before the 1960's the average medical doctor totally ignored cholesterol unless it exceeded 300. When the anti-cholesterol campaign ramped up the volume and became impossible to ignore, the medical establishment started to pay attention. Then, anything above 250 was considered a problem, and it was generally recommended that people should avoid eating too many eggs or too much meat because of the "risk of heart disease from cholesterol intake". We now know that eating cholesterol in diet has nothing to do with raising blood cholesterol since your liver makes an appropriate amount of cholesterol no matter how much you eat. Quite simply, if you eat less cholesterol in the diet your liver will make more to make up the difference and on the other hand, if you eat more cholesterol in the diet your liver will make less to compensate for the decreased need. Has your medical doctor told you not to eat eggs because your cholesterol is "too high"? The *Journal of the American*

Medical Association stated, "Research shows that there is absolutely no connection between eating eggs and the risk of heart disease or stroke in either men or women." (*JAMA* 1999; 281(15): 1387-94) Your liver makes about 2,000 mg. of cholesterol per day. Is your liver trying to kill you from heart disease? Certainly not.

Back to our cholesterol history. Interestingly, it wasn't the medical profession that was spearheading this anti-cholesterol movement; it was the processed food industry, lead in particular by the seed oil industry. Archer Daniels Midland wanted to sell an ocean of soybean oil, and thus lead the charge against cholesterol in particular and saturated fat in general. Coconut and palm oils were banned from importation, and everyone "knew" that margarine (an extremely dangerous partially hydrogenated seed oil) was going to save our nation from what was sure to have been an epidemic of cardiovascular disease from eating the dreaded saturated fat. The trouble is stearic acid, an 18 carbon saturated fat, one of the most abundant fats in steak doesn't raise LDL cholesterol levels. On the other hand, all the omega-6 seed oils such as soybean, sunflower, safflower, peanut and corn oil tend to promote the formation of inflammatory chemicals called prostaglandins.

Then statin drugs happened and the rest is what we have today. The all-out war against cholesterol has been waged for over 25 years. The intensity of that war has not waned in the least despite the fact that for at least five years now it has been known that cholesterol is not (never has been, and never will be) a primary risk factor for cardiovascular disease!

Who decided what cholesterol levels are healthy or harmful? In 2004, the U.S. government's National Cholesterol Education Program (NCEP) panel advised those at risk for heart disease to reduce their LDL cholesterol to specific, very low levels. Before 2004, a 130 milligram LDL cholesterol level was considered healthy. The updated guidelines, however, recommended levels of less than 100, or even less than 70 for patients at very high risk. Keep in mind that these extremely low targets often require multiple cholesterol-lowering drugs to achieve since this is going against what the body's natural mechanisms are trying to achieve. However, in 2006 a review in the *Annals of Internal Medicine* found that there was insufficient evidence to support the target numbers outlined by the panel. The authors of the review were unable to find research providing evidence that achieving a specific LDL target level was important in and of itself, and found that the studies attempting to do so suffered from major flaws. Several of the scientists who helped develop the guidelines even admitted that the scientific evidence supporting the less than 70 recommendation was not very strong. So how did these excessively low cholesterol guidelines come about?

Eight of the nine doctors on the panel that developed the new cholesterol guidelines had been making money from the drug companies that manufacture statin cholesterol-lowering drugs. These are the same drugs that the new guidelines suddenly created a huge new market for in the United States. Coincidence? Probably not. Let's face it. Cholesterol drugs are a cash cow for the pharmaceutical industry. Lipitor™ is one of the best selling drugs of all time and has close to a 4,700% markup in price. Statin medications account for 6.5% of all drug sales in the United States to the tune of $12.5 billion dollars. (And that was back in 2005) No wonder it is so hard to change guidelines. Sadly, despite the finding that there is absolutely NO evidence to show that lowering your LDL cholesterol to 100 or below is good for you, what do you think the American Heart Association still recommends? That's right. Lowering your LDL cholesterol levels to less than 100. Remember, you almost always need a medication to get the LDL level that low.

Are there dangers to having low cholesterol? You bet. If you look at the physiology and metabolism of cholesterol you will begin to understand how important this substance is. Not only is cholesterol vital for all cell membrane health as discussed earlier, but it is also a precursor for many other critical hormones and nutrients such as vitamin D, bile salts for fat digestion, and steroid hormones such as progesterone, estrogen and testosterone. Anti-oxidants are also ferried in the body on lipoproteins so low cholesterol will lead to increased oxidation or aging. One of the more well known ways this happens is through the suppression of formation of co-enzyme Q10 or CoQ10. CoQ10 is an important co-factor and anti-oxidant in the membranes of our mitochondria, the little furnaces that make the energy currency of life called ATP. One of the problems is our little mitochondrial furnaces are a little sloppy when they make ATP and some of the free radicals produced in this process leak out and lead to cell damage. If the proper anti-oxidant defenses are not in place to mop up these damaging molecules such as CoQ10, this can lead to serious disease.

Blood levels of CoQ10 decrease with age, high blood pressure or hypertension, statin use, diabetes and atherosclerosis. A CoQ10 deficiency can lead to muscle pain (a common side effect to taking statins), angina, hypertension, accelerated aging and heart disease. CoQ10 is also vital to the formation of two of the most common connective tissues in the body, elastin and collagen. Side effects of CoQ10 deficiency in this area include muscle wasting that may lead to weakness and severe back pain, heart failure (remember the heart is a muscle), neuropathy, and inflammation of the tendons and ligaments, often leading to rupture.

Muscle pain and weakness from statins is thought to occur since these drugs activate the atrogin-1 gene, which plays a key role in muscle atrophy.

One statin, Baycol™, was withdrawn from the market because it was linked to 52 deaths from rhabdomyolysis or muscle death and over 1,100 cases of muscle weakness. The other statins still pose a rare risk for this disorder, especially at doses of 80 mg. per day.

Since cholesterol is vital to the nervous system it should be no surprise to find significant side effects involving nerves. A Denmark study that evaluated 500,000 patients found that people who took statins were more likely to develop polyneuropathy or nerve damage. Taking statins for one year raised the risk of nerve damage by about 15% - about one case for every 2,200 patients. For those who took statins for more than two or more years, the additional risk rose to 26%. (*Southern Medical Journal* 96(12): 1265-1267, December 2003 and *Neurology* 2002 May 14; 58(9): 1321-2)

There is also a possible association statins and an increased risk of Lou Gehrig's disease (amyotrophic lateral sclerosis)(*Drug Safety* Volume 30, No. 6 2007: 515-525) as well as cognitive impairment and memory loss. Remember, a large part of the brain is made up of cholesterol.

It should be a big tip-off to the danger of a drug if doctors must monitor your blood every 3 months to check for liver damage.

Even William Castelli, M.D., a former director of the Framingham Heart Study noted :

"People with low cholesterol (lower than 200) suffer nearly 40% of all heart attacks."

This means predicting who would have a heart attack by using cholesterol levels was about as good as flipping a coin.

More disturbing, people with cholesterol less than 180 have three times the incidence of strokes as the general population.

To throw another wrench into the machine, a study done by Gilman et al. and published in the December 24, 1997 *Journal of the American Medical Association* found that the more saturated fat you eat, the less likely you are to suffer a stroke. It goes on to state that polyunsaturated fats (the seed oils we have been told to eat) have no protective effect. Best of all, this study actually was able to quantify the protective effect of saturated fats. **The risk of stroke decreases by 15% for every 3% increase in saturated fat intake.**

One last study to bring home this point which was published in *Medicine and Science in Sports and Exercise* Volume 29, 1997. The subjects of this study were elite male and female endurance athletes, who were placed alternately on a high fat diet and then a low fat diet. On a high saturated fat diet the patients maintained low body fat, normal weight, normal blood pressure, normal resting heart rate, normal triglycerides and normal serum cholesterol levels. All their fitness and training parameters were maintained at the elite level. When put on the low fat (high complex carbohydrate) diet, however, it was found that the low fat diet negated many of the beneficial effects that exercise is expected to produce. The athletes experienced measurable decline in athletic performance. Most interesting, however, was the fat that the subjects on the low fat diet actually suffered a significant drop in HDL cholesterol along with higher triglycerides (both of these situations are significant CVD risk factors). We can see this from an article in the journal *Circulation* October 21, 1997 which stated: The 25% of the population with the highest triglyceride to HDL ratio has 16 times more heart related events than the 25% whose ratios were the lowest.

There is ample evidence linking low cholesterol to depression and suicide.

- Several studies show that among older adults, those with lowered cholesterol are more likely to suffer from depression. (*BMJ*, 1996: 312: 1289-99)
- Those with low cholesterol are three times more likely to suffer from depression as normal adults. (Same as above)

- The *British Medical Journal* published research showing that the lower the cholesterol, the more severe the depression. (Same as above)
- Low cholesterol levels are also linked to an increased risk of committing suicide. In one study, reported in the *British Medical Journal*, showed that of the 300 people who had committed suicide, ALL had low cholesterol levels. (*BMJ*, 1995: 310: 1632-36)
- Men whose cholesterol levels are lowered through prescription medications double their chances of committing suicide. (*BMJ*, 1996: 313: 649-64)

And What About Women?

The *Journal of the American Medical Association* reports that there is no evidence linking high cholesterol levels in women with heart disease. (*JAMA*, 1995: 274(14): 1152-58

In case you missed that last sentence I will repeat it. Total cholesterol levels for women have been shown to be meaningless! How many women are put on statins?

In addition, Dr. Thomas Newman of the University of California at San Fransisco, who has written extensively on cholesterol and heart disease, reports that cholesterol medications are less beneficial to women and may even increase their risk of death. (*NEJM,* 1996: 334(20) 1334)

How Effective Are Cholesterol Medications Anyway?

In statistics there is a number known as the NNT or number needed to treat. The NNT answers the question: How many people have to take a particular drug to avoid one incidence of a medical issue (such as a heart attack)? For example, if a drug had an NNT of 50 for heart attacks, then 50 people would have to take the drug in order to prevent one heart attack. If you use the NNT you get a slightly different picture regarding the pharmaceutical companies 'miracle' drugs.

Let's take Lipitor™, Pfizer's blockbuster drug, for instance. It is the most prescribed cholesterol medication in the world with over 26 million Americans taking it. According to Lipitor's™ own website, the drug is clinically proven to lower 'bad' cholesterol 39 - 60%, depending on the dose. Sounds great, right? Well, *BusinessWeek* actually did an excellent story on this very topic and found the REAL numbers right on Pfizer's own newspaper ad for Lipitor™ Upon first glance, the ad boasts that Lipitor™ reduces heart attacks by 36%. However, there is an asterisk. When you follow the asterisk, you find the following in much smaller type:

"That means in a large clinical study, 3% of patients taking a sugar pill or placebo had a heart attack compared to 2% of patients taking Lipitor™"

What this means is that for every 100 people who took the drug over 3.3 years, three people on placebos, and two people on Lipitor™, had heart attacks. That means that taking Lipitor™ resulted in just one fewer heart attack per 100 people. The NNT, in this case, is 100. One hundred people have to take Lipitor™ for more than three years to prevent one heart attack. The other 99 people have just dished out hundreds of dollars and increased their risk of a multitude of side effects for nothing.

How about other drugs like Zetia™ and Vytorin™? Early in 2008, it came out that Zetia™, which works by inhibiting absorption of cholesterol from the intestines, and Vytorin™, which is a combination of Zetia™ and Zocor™ (a statin drug), do not work. It was only after the results of a trial by the drugs' manufacturers, Merck and Schering-Plough, were released that this fact was discovered. Incidentally, this was discovered AFTER the drugs acquired close to 20% of the U.S. market for cholesterol lowering drugs. This was also after close to 1 million prescriptions for the drugs were being written each week in the United States, bringing in close to $4 billion in 2007.

Zetia™ does reduce cholesterol by 15 - 20%, but trials failed to show a reduction in heart attacks or strokes, or that it reduces plaques in arteries that can lead to heart problems. Isn't this what most people are taking the drug for?

The trial by the drug's makers, which studied whether Zetia™ could reduce the growth of plaques, found that *plaques grew nearly twice as fast* in patients taking Zetia™ along with Zocor™ (Vytorin™) than in those taking Zocor™ alone. That is not good news.

So What Causes Heart Attacks and Strokes?

If it isn't cholesterol and saturated fat, then what does cause these major killers? It turns out that these are inflammatory diseases at the core. Chronic inflammation is the overproduction of certain cytokines or cell chemical messengers which lead to the actual tissue damage. If you look at laboratory values of cholesterol, this is analogous to the engine light in your car. When cholesterol levels increase it means that the body is undergoing some kind of metabolic stress. It doesn't tell you what it is, just like the engine light doesn't tell you what the car problem is. The underlying cause needs to be addressed. For instance, rising total cholesterol and LDL cholesterol is typically an indicator of dysglycemia or blood sugar problems. It could also be from adrenal gland dysfunction (your fight of flight gland), infection, thyroid issues, food sensitivities or many other causes but usually blood sugar is one of the first things to address. Here is a list of the major factors in developing heart disease:

- Excess dietary polyunsaturated fats. These are the fats found in vegetable oils like soybean, corn, sunflower and safflower. Since they are unsaturated, which means they have many double bonds which are prone to attack from oxygen, they go rancid very easily. Excess polyunsaturates have been shown to contribute to heart disease, cancer, weight gain and many other health problems. On the other side of the coin is the lack of the so-called omega-3 fats which are your fish oils, flax oils, krill oils and linolenic acid from green plants. These oils lead to the anti-inflammatory prostaglandins mentioned earlier.
- Excess dietary carbohydrates leading to excess insulin. Insulin is an extremely inflammatory protein which has been found to be responsible for atherosclerotic lesions. Controlling insulin levels should be an important objective towards averting a heart attack. Excess insulin has also been responsible for vasoconstriction or narrowing of blood vessels and blood clotting, two more factors that contribute to arterial blockages.
- Thyroid insufficiency
- Excess estrogen which leads to increased clotting risk
- Testosterone insuffiency
- Excess catecholamines (epinephrine or adrenaline, norepinephrine and dopamine).

Studies have found that the increased secretion of stress hormones when someone is angry (epinephrine, norepinephrine and dopamine) can damage the endothelium, a layer of thin, flattened cells that line the arteries and can accelerate the development of atherosclerosis. These hormones can also disrupt the electrical rhythm of the heart as well as increase platelet adhesion. Platelets assist in normal, healthy blood clotting, but they can also adhere to sites of endothelium damage, which can lead to blockage.

➢ Excess cortisol. Cortisol regulates your blood sugar. High levels of cortisol can damage the hippocampus of the brain - this is the short term memory and learning center.

➢ Oxidative stress to the heart and arteries. Apples turn brown, butter turns rancid, iron rusts. All of these are everyday signs of oxidative stress - destruction caused by free radical molecules. None of these examples compare to what these unstable molecules can do inside the body, especially to cells of the brain and vessels of the heart.

➢ Magnesium deficiency with excess calcium or other trace mineral deficiencies.

What are the Clinical Indicators of Cardiovascular Disease?

➢ Cardiac arrhythmia. These can be picked up on ECG or other standard cardiac testing.

➢ Elevated triglycerides (particularly an elevated triglyceride to HDL ratio). Elevated blood levels of triglycerides, but not cholesterol, have been associated with an impaired fibrinolytic system (blood clotting system). Fibrinogen is also a good test to discern an increased potential for a heart attack. Studies have implicated triglycerides in the progression of coronary atherosclerosis.

➢ Elevated homocysteine. Homocysteine acts as a molecular abrasive by scraping the inner layer of blood vessels. Therefore, high levels of homocysteine have been correlated with damaged endothelium and the formation of atherosclerotic lesions. One study found that men with extremely high homocysteine levels were three times more likely to have an associated myocardial infarction.

➢ Elevated insulin. Hyperinsulinemia with normal blood glucose is a factor associated with the etiology of hyperlipidemias and is an independent risk factor for heart disease.

➢ Elevated cortisol levels. High levels of cortisol are associated with hypertension, and, interestingly, it has been found that simply having a family history of hypertension predisposes an individual to exaggerated cortisol secretion in response to stress. Patients with heart disease exhibit higher cortisol levels than do controls.

➢ Elevated estrogen in respect to progesterone.

➢ Low testosterone in men. Chronically low testosterone levels may actually precede coronary artery disease and thrombosis (clot formation) whereas higher levels of testosterone have been found to offer men greater than 5-fold protection against atherosclerotic coronary artery disease. British cardiologists in the *Quarterly Journal of Medicine* found that normal physiological levels of testosterone may protect against the development of hyperlipidemia, hyperinsulinism and hypertension.

➢ High testosterone in women. Although testosterone may produce strong beneficial effects on an amazingly wide array of CVD risks in men, high levels of testosterone exert a detrimental influence on cardiovascular health in women. This is usually a consequence of high blood sugar and insulin resistance.

➢ Lipid peroxides. These are the products of chemical damage produced by oxygen free radicals to the lipid components of cell membranes. High levels of lipid peroxides are associated with cancer, heart disease, stroke and aging.

➢ Elevated C-reactive protein. Inflammation is a crucial factor in the pathogenesis of atherothrombosis. C-reactive protein is a non-specific marker associated with the production of inflammatory cytokines. These cytokines appear to encourage coagulation and damage vascular endothelium (the delicate lining of blood vessels), increasing the potential threat to cardiovascular health.

➢ Mineral deficiencies, especially magnesium and zinc.

➢ Fatty acid imbalance usually too much omega-6 fats and not enough omega-3 as described earlier. (Remember, fats make up 70% of the brain)

➢ Thyroid dysfunction

As unbelievable as it may seem, we have a condition that kills more than 50% of all people, yet most doctors are entirely ignorant of the causes of this condition. The good news is all these indicators can be monitored and can be dealt with using a lifestyle/nutritional approach.

How Should Cholesterol Issues Be Addressed?

Since an abnormal cholesterol panel is an indicator physiological stress in the body, the underlying causes of this stress should be addressed. The four basic pillars of functional medicine involved in controlling the inflammatory process are:

- ✓ Anemias
- ✓ Blood sugar/adrenal issues
- ✓ Liver/gastrointestinal issues
- ✓ Fatty acid metabolism

There is one other situation that trumps the above four pillars and that is an autoimmune condition. Autoimmunity is a state wherein your immune system recognizes one or more of your own tissues as foreign and attempts to destroy them. This process drives the other four pillars, therefore, autoimmunity becomes the primary problem to support.

Monitoring should ALWAYS be done with the appropriate laboratory testing.

If you are like most patients, you have been indoctrinated by the well-meaning medical community that cholesterol is the evil that causes heart disease. We have been mislead to believe that if we monitor cholesterol levels and avoid the foods alleged to raise cholesterol, you will be safe from America's number one killer.

Each patient has unique genetics and risk factors so a recovery program requires a health professional that understands the complexities of functional medicine. This is what sets myself and other functional medicine practitioners apart. Please, do not try to do this alone!

Remember, chronic inflammation is usually silent. Don't let an ambulance ride to the emergency room be the first time you think about your risk factors for heart disease. Take the steps towards true prevention!

For questions, contact Dr. Miller at:

drmiller@miller-chiro.com

16675352R00014

Made in the USA
Charleston, SC
05 January 2013